Phrasebook for Paramedics

A concise lexicon for efficient communication in emergency situations

Arden Hendricks

Table of Contents

1 Chapter 1: Initial Assessment

The initial assessment is paramount. It dictates the course of treatment and, quite possibly, the patient's outcome. Begin by rapidly establishing the scene's safety—yours and your team's, as well as the patient's. Assess any immediate threats, such as fire, traffic, or hazardous materials, before approaching. This crucial first step safeguards everyone involved.

Next, immediately assess the patient's level of consciousness. Use the AVPU scale—Alert, Verbal response, Pain response, Unresponsive—a simple yet powerful tool for rapid triage. This initial assessment will guide your subsequent actions, dictating the urgency and nature of your interventions. A patient who is alert and oriented will require a different approach than one who's unresponsive.

Vitals are the foundation of your assessment. Begin with the ABCs—Airway, Breathing, Circulation—checking for patency, respiratory rate and quality, and the presence of a pulse. Note the skin's color, temperature, and moisture, which can often provide vital clues about the patient's condition. Don't forget to monitor oxygen saturation using a pulse oximeter, and be prepared to initiate supplemental oxygen if necessary. These seemingly simple checks will reveal crucial information about your patient's physiological state. This will help you to avoid mistakes. Remember

that observing the patient while conducting these assessments will provide additional insights into his or her overall condition.
A thorough history is critical. Ask the patient, or those present, about the chief complaint—what prompted the call for help? This sets the direction of your entire assessment. Don't be afraid to ask probing questions to get a clearer picture. Was there an injury? A sudden onset of symptoms? Prior medical history is also critical; find out about any pre-existing conditions, allergies, and current medications. Gather information carefully and methodically; a comprehensive patient history is essential for effective treatment. Consider using memory aids—MIST, SAMPLE, or OPQRST—to assist with your questioning.
The SAMPLE mnemonic—Symptoms, Allergies, Medications, Past medical history, Last meal, Events leading to the illness or injury—is incredibly helpful for collecting a patient history. It provides a structured framework that helps to minimize the possibility of neglecting vital information. Remember, accuracy and completeness are paramount. Listen attentively. Ask clarifying questions. Your ability to elicit accurate information directly impacts your ability to make sound clinical judgments and provide appropriate care.
Gathering an accurate history can sometimes be tricky. Patients in distress may be unable to provide comprehensive details. In such cases, family members, friends, or bystanders become invaluable sources of information. Don't overlook this information as crucial context. Even seemingly minor details might prove to be significant clues to understanding the patient's condition. Combine information from various sources to create the fullest possible picture.
Always be mindful of your surroundings; the environment may provide further insight into the cause of the emergency. Was there a fall? A motor vehicle accident? A potential exposure to toxins? The scene may offer critical clues. Document all observations carefully; it helps to avoid potential future uncertainties.
Remember, the initial assessment is not just a checklist; it's a dy-

namic process. You must continuously reassess the patient as your understanding of their condition evolves. Vitals can change rapidly, and new symptoms might arise. This continuous evaluation and monitoring ensures you remain flexible and are ready to adapt your treatment plan. Never hesitate to adjust your approach as the situation dictates. Your initial assessment creates the foundation upon which all subsequent actions are built.
This initial assessment sets the stage for the rest of the emergency care. A comprehensive and accurate assessment, performed with precision and care, makes a real difference in the patient's outcome. Take your time, but always remember efficiency is critical. A thorough assessment will significantly impact the effectiveness of all subsequent actions taken. Your actions must be thorough, well-thought-out and precisely executed. Accurate observation and well-phrased questions will provide the best basis for treatment. The well-being of the patient depends on the quality of this initial assessment.

1.1 Vitals & Signs

Precisely measuring vital signs forms the bedrock of any effective emergency response. A seemingly insignificant fluctuation in heart rate, for instance, could signal impending cardiac arrest, while a subtle drop in blood pressure might indicate internal bleeding. Mastering the techniques to accurately assess these indicators is paramount; it's the difference between reacting appropriately and potentially overlooking a life-threatening condition. Remember the importance of regular calibration of your equipment; inaccurate readings are as detrimental as missed readings.
Your initial assessment always begins with a quick visual scan, evaluating the patient's overall appearance—are they conscious and alert, or are they exhibiting signs of distress? Observe their breathing pattern: Is it shallow, labored, or absent? Note their skin color—pallor can suggest shock, cyanosis indicates a lack of

oxygen, and flushed skin might point to fever or other conditions. This seemingly simple first step informs your next actions. The speed and accuracy at which you visually assess the situation will often determine the success of the intervention.

Measuring the pulse is a basic skill, yet crucial to mastering. Feel for the radial pulse at the wrist, but if you can't locate it, try the carotid pulse in the neck. Count the beats for a full minute, noting the rhythm—is it regular or irregular, strong or weak? A rapid pulse can indicate shock, anxiety, or fever; a slow pulse might signal a heart condition or medication effect. Take the time, don't rush this vital step. You need to accurately capture this data. Documentation, clear and concise, is as critical as the measurement itself.

Blood pressure measurement is equally vital. Knowing how to properly use a sphygmomanometer is non-negotiable. Inflate the cuff until the pulse disappears, then slowly release, noting the point at which you hear the first clear sound (systolic pressure) and the point at which the sound disappears completely (diastolic pressure). Record these numbers precisely and systematically in your patient's chart. A sudden drop in blood pressure, for instance, is a critical indicator that requires immediate attention. It's important to be aware that factors like patient position and cuff size impact accuracy.

Respiratory rate is another key vital sign. Observe the patient's chest movements over a full minute. Count the number of breaths per minute, noting their depth and regularity. Shallow, rapid breathing could signal respiratory distress, while slow or irregular breathing can indicate other underlying medical issues. Never underestimate the importance of observation; sometimes subtle differences in breathing patterns are the only visible clues to a serious medical problem. Always observe and record the breath sounds, searching for any abnormalities like wheezing or rattling.

Temperature assessment is often overlooked. Though not always immediately life-threatening, a high or low temperature can significantly impact a patient's condition and guides your subse-

quent decisions. Use a reliable thermometer, either oral or axillary (armpit), depending on the patient's cooperation and overall state. It's essential to have a clear understanding of normal ranges and deviations that may signal underlying illness or infection. Consider the impact of environmental factors on body temperature in the field.
Finally, always remember the importance of Oxygen Saturation (SpO2) monitoring. Using a pulse oximeter, a non-invasive method of measuring blood oxygen levels is crucial. Low SpO2 readings highlight the urgent need for supplemental oxygen. The readings, coupled with respiratory rate and other observations, can provide a comprehensive picture of the patient's respiratory status. You must always understand the limitations of a pulse oximeter; it doesn't replace a thorough clinical assessment.
The accurate and timely assessment of vital signs is not just a procedure; it is a crucial skill set that significantly impacts patient outcomes. Consistent practice and a methodical approach will build your proficiency. Remember, clear and precise communication of these findings to the receiving hospital is just as important as the data collection itself, ensuring the best continuity of care for the patient. Consider the potential impact of your errors; a misinterpretation can have critical consequences. Never compromise on precision or accuracy, even under pressure. Your expertise in this critical area will help save lives.

1.2 Patient History

Gathering a patient's history is the cornerstone of effective emergency care. It's not simply a checklist; it's a crucial conversation, a narrative pieced together to understand the unfolding emergency. This process helps you build a complete picture of their condition, enabling you to prioritize interventions and ultimately, improve outcomes. Effective communication and active listening are paramount.

The initial interaction sets the tone. Your demeanor should convey calm confidence, reassuring the patient while allowing for honest and open communication. Start by introducing yourself clearly, identifying your role, and outlining the purpose of your questioning. This approach fosters trust and encourages the patient to cooperate. Avoid medical jargon; use plain language they can easily understand.

Don't underestimate the power of the chief complaint. This is the patient's statement describing their primary concern. It provides your first clue, guiding the subsequent line of questioning. Listen carefully, noting not only the words themselves, but also the tone of voice, facial expressions, and overall body language. These nonverbal cues often reveal additional information that might not be explicitly stated. For example, a patient complaining of chest pain might subtly clutch their chest or exhibit shallow breathing. This combination of verbal and nonverbal cues paints a more complete picture than either alone.

Thoroughly exploring the history of present illness (HPI) requires a systematic approach. Employ open-ended questions like "Can you tell me more about your symptoms?" to encourage detailed narratives. Follow up with clarifying questions, such as "When did the symptoms begin?" "Where is the pain located?" and "What makes the pain better or worse?" A chronological timeline of events can prove incredibly valuable.

Don't overlook the importance of past medical history. Knowing about existing conditions—heart disease, diabetes, allergies—significantly impacts treatment decisions. Inquire about hospitalizations, surgeries, and current medications, including dosage and frequency. Even seemingly minor details can have significant implications. For instance, an allergy to a specific medication could be life-threatening if inadvertently administered. This aspect requires meticulous attention to detail. Never assume anything.

Allergies, both medication and environmental, demand clear and direct questioning. Document each allergy precisely, noting the specific allergen and the nature of the reaction. This information is critical for avoiding potentially fatal reactions. Consider allergies not only to medications but also to environmental factors like pollen, animal dander, or certain foods. These allergies can sometimes trigger unexpected medical responses. Remember to record reactions; a simple "rash" is less informative than "anaphylactic shock".

While you're focused on immediate symptoms, remember to gather a comprehensive social history. This is an often-overlooked area, yet crucial for understanding the context of the patient's situation. Inquire about lifestyle factors—smoking, alcohol or drug use, occupation, and living situation. This data might highlight potential risk factors or provide clues relevant to their condition. For example, someone who works in a dusty environment might experience respiratory problems. This seemingly insignificant detail, in the context of other gathered information, might indicate an occupational hazard instead of an acute condition. Every detail is a piece of a larger puzzle.

Finally, always remember the importance of family history. Understanding whether a patient's family has a history of heart disease, cancer, or other genetic predispositions can give you valuable insight into their current condition and risk factors. This knowledge aids in your assessment and allows you to prioritize specific areas of examination and intervention. Keep your questions precise; however, don't hesitate to probe deeper if necessary. A thorough family history provides critical contextual information about hereditary traits and potential vulnerabilities. Always maintain sensitivity during this part of the interaction; family history can be emotionally charged for the patient. Your empathy and professionalism will facilitate cooperation. Remember, your comprehensive and patient approach is essential for delivering optimal emergency care and improving patient outcomes. This structured approach ensures nothing is overlooked. Taking the time for thorough patient history collection ensures the patient receives the most appropriate and effective emergency treatment.

2 Chapter 2: Trauma Response

Effective trauma response hinges on rapid assessment and decisive action. Time is of the essence; every second counts in preventing further injury and preserving life. Your initial survey should focus on identifying life-threatening conditions – massive bleeding, airway obstruction, or signs of shock – addressing these immediately before moving on to other injuries. This prioritization is crucial.

Control of external bleeding is paramount. Direct pressure, applied firmly and continuously over the wound, is the first line of defense. Elevate the injured limb if possible, further aiding in reducing blood flow. For severe, uncontrolled bleeding, a tourniquet may be necessary. Remember to document the exact time of tourniquet application – this is vital information for subsequent medical care. Never underestimate the power of simple, direct pressure. If the bleeding continues, and the patient's condition deteriorates rapidly despite your efforts, additional measures will be necessary.

Fracture management involves stabilizing the injured area to prevent further damage and pain. Splinting techniques vary depending on the location and type of fracture. Your primary goal is immobilization above and below the fracture site, minimizing movement. Always check for distal pulses to ensure adequate blood circulation after splinting. Improper splinting can restrict blood flow and cause additional injury. Use appropriate padding to prevent pressure sores and ensure comfortable positioning. Pay close attention to the patient's overall condition.

Recognizing and treating shock is a critical skill. Shock is a life-threatening condition characterized by inadequate blood flow to the body's organs. Common signs include pale, clammy skin, rapid weak pulse, rapid breathing, and altered mental status. Treatment involves maintaining a patent airway, administering supplemental oxygen, controlling external bleeding, and keeping the patient warm. In cases of suspected hypovolemic shock (due to blood loss), intravenous fluids may be necessary. Remember that timely and aggressive intervention is critical in improving the patient's chances of survival. Early recognition and treatment often mean the difference between life and death.

Understanding the physiological responses to trauma is essential for effective intervention. The body's initial reaction involves a surge of adrenaline, preparing it to cope with the emergency. This can manifest as increased heart rate, blood pressure, and respiration. However, prolonged or severe trauma can overwhelm the body's compensatory mechanisms, leading to shock. Your knowledge of these physiological processes allows you to anticipate potential complications and act accordingly. It's not just about immediate treatment; it's about recognizing the patterns and understanding the implications of the body's reaction to trauma.

Trauma patients often experience pain and anxiety. Providing reassurance and emotional support, while maintaining professional distance, is crucial. Clear and concise communication can significantly alleviate a patient's distress. Explain procedures clearly, answering questions honestly and patiently, even if the answers are difficult. Remember that trauma patients often suffer from a cascade of physical and psychological reactions, and your empathy plays a pivotal role. Your demeanor and empathy can influence the patient's experience.

Always remember that you're not just treating injuries; you're managing a whole person. Be mindful of the patient's overall condition; don't get tunnel vision on a single injury. A thorough assessment, including vital signs monitoring, is necessary throughout the process. Reassess regularly. The patient's condition can change rapidly. Continual monitoring is key to detecting any deterioration and initiating prompt intervention. A holistic approach ensures optimal patient care.

After stabilization, careful transport to a definitive care facility is critical. Ensure that all necessary information is accurately documented and communicated to the receiving hospital. Include the mechanisms of injury, interventions performed, and any significant findings during your assessment. Accurate and concise documentation is vital for continuity of care, potentially saving the patient's life.

Accurate communication is paramount, not only with your team but also with the patient and their family. Explain your actions clearly. A calm, reassuring manner can significantly reduce anxiety in a stressful situation. The power of effective communication should never be underestimated. Remember, your actions speak louder than words, but you must back them up with clear and concise language. Effective communication is an essential skill for any paramedic. Always remember the ethical and legal aspects that are inherent to providing quality care.

2.1 Bleeding Control

Direct pressure remains the cornerstone of bleeding control. Apply firm, consistent pressure directly to the wound using a clean dressing. Elevate the injured limb above the heart, if possible, to reduce blood flow. Continue applying pressure until bleeding stops or professional medical assistance arrives. Remember, consistent, direct pressure is paramount; don't repeatedly check for bleeding as this disrupts the clotting process. Your actions in these initial moments can be life-saving.

Effective communication is critical, even during frantic situations. Clearly articulate the severity of the bleeding to dispatch, providing details such as the location, type, and estimated volume of blood loss. This allows emergency services to prepare appropriately and potentially expedite their response, offering better chances for survival. This concise, clear communication is your primary tool; use it efficiently. Your words become a lifeline.

Tourniquets, a last resort for severe, life-threatening bleeding, demand precise application. Apply it two to three inches above the wound, tightening until bleeding stops. Once applied, mark the time of application on the tourniquet itself with a marker, pen, or even a watch strap. This critical piece of information is vital for hospital staff to manage the patient's care effectively, minimizing limb damage. Never loosen a tourniquet unless instructed by a qualified medical professional, even if the patient requests it.

Hemostatic dressings, which contain clotting agents, can significantly accelerate the clotting process. These advanced dressings, when applied directly to the wound, absorb blood and actively promote clot formation. Their effectiveness is particularly pronounced in cases of arterial bleeding, where rapid blood loss is a significant threat. This option, though not always available, offers a more effective alternative to basic dressings in severe cases. Proper application is key for optimal effectiveness.

Internal bleeding presents a unique challenge, often masked by symptoms like abdominal pain, shock, and reduced level of consciousness. Recognizing the subtle signs is crucial for timely intervention. Immediate transport to the hospital is essential, as internal bleeding requires more invasive procedures. While you can't directly stop internal bleeding, your careful observation and quick action can facilitate appropriate care at a medical facility. These seemingly minor symptoms should not be overlooked.

For severe head injuries, focus on maintaining an open airway and preventing further trauma. Control external bleeding with gentle pressure, avoiding unnecessary movement of the head and neck. Suspect internal bleeding and act accordingly; rapid transport is a crucial part of their care. You must carefully monitor their breathing and consciousness; this type of injury necessitates swift response.

Remember, assessing the wound and the overall patient condition is paramount. It's not just about controlling the bleeding but also about maintaining the patient's airway, breathing, and circulation. Your role involves a comprehensive approach; the bleeding is just one piece of the puzzle. The speed and efficacy of your assessment directly impact the outcome.

Beyond the physical techniques, emotional support plays a vital role. Reassurance to the injured person and bystanders is equally important. Your calm demeanor and clear instructions can help alleviate anxiety and promote cooperation, making the entire process more efficient and potentially saving lives. Remember, a calm demeanor benefits everyone.

Keep in mind, the information provided here is a guideline, not a replacement for formal medical training. Regular refresher courses and continued professional development are essential for all paramedics. Maintaining proficiency in bleeding control techniques is not only a professional responsibility but also a critical aspect of saving lives. This skill needs constant refining and honing for effective practice. Regular training will only enhance your skill set and potentially make a life-altering impact.

Documenting your actions in detail is critical. Record the time of the incident, the location, the type of bleeding, the interventions performed, and the patient's response to treatment. Accurate and concise documentation is not merely a procedural requirement; it's integral to providing high quality care and minimizing liability. It's a safety net for you, and a guarantee of comprehensive care for your patient. Remember, detailed documentation protects everyone involved.

Finally, always prioritize the safety of yourself and your team. Approach all bleeding control situations cautiously, ensuring your safety, and that of your crew. Follow established protocols and guidelines, and don't hesitate to request additional support if needed. Safety in practice is non-negotiable. It's about protecting both the patient and yourself in the line of duty. It's an essential part of your overall professional responsibility.

2.2 Fracture Management

Fractures, breaks in the bone, demand immediate and skillful attention. Improper handling can worsen the injury, leading to increased pain, nerve damage, and even life-threatening complications. Therefore, your primary goal is to stabilize the fracture, minimizing movement and preventing further harm. Remember, patient comfort is paramount, and your actions should reflect that. A calm and reassuring demeanor can greatly ease their distress during what is undoubtedly a painful experience.

Assessing the injury starts with a visual inspection. Note the location of the fracture, any visible deformity, and the presence of any open wounds. Ask the patient about their pain level, using a standardized pain scale to aid in objective assessment and tracking. Don't forget to check for distal pulses – feeling for blood flow beyond the injury site is crucial in identifying any potential compromise to circulation. A lack of pulse indicates a serious complication that requires immediate attention and further interventions, potentially involving vascular surgeons. The patient's skin color and temperature also provide valuable clues; pallor or coolness may suggest compromised circulation requiring careful reassessment and a more thorough approach to managing the issue. Proper documentation of these observations is essential, building a clear and accurate record of the patient's condition for subsequent medical professionals.

Immobilization is key. Your choice of splinting technique will depend on the location and type of fracture. A simple fracture of a forearm might be adequately splinted using a rigid splint, ensuring it's padded to prevent pressure sores. For more complex injuries, such as a suspected pelvic fracture, a more comprehensive approach is vital; stabilization might necessitate the use of a backboard and careful handling during transport. Remember the principles of splinting: immobilize the joint above and below the fracture site. This minimizes movement and helps reduce the risk of further trauma to the already compromised bone and surrounding tissue. When in doubt, err on the side of caution and utilize more extensive immobilization techniques.

Pain management is an integral part of fracture care. Administer analgesics as appropriate, following local protocols and considering the patient's overall condition. Remember, the goal is to provide sufficient pain relief without compromising their respiration or awareness. Your communication with the patient is also crucial; they may require reassurance and explanation throughout the process. It's important to convey your competence while empathizing with their pain. A simple act of holding their hand and speaking in a calm, steady voice can make a considerable difference to their comfort and cooperation during transport to definitive care. Even seemingly minor gestures can be quite effective.

Transportation requires careful planning. Ensure the patient is securely immobilized and transported in the most appropriate vehicle for their condition. Clear communication with the receiving hospital is vital, including the nature and severity of the injury, the interventions provided, and the patient's vital signs. Providing comprehensive information streamlines the handover process and allows the receiving medical team to prepare accordingly for receiving the patient. Any delay in reporting can result in less efficient management and potentially compromise the patient's condition further. Timely and effective communication is vital.

Beyond the immediate response, remember that your role extends to the documentation aspect. Your detailed report forms the basis for subsequent treatment decisions. Include all relevant information: the mechanism of injury, your assessment findings, the interventions you implemented, the patient's response, and their vital signs throughout your involvement. Precision in recording pain scores, pulse checks, and other significant indicators is crucial for the ongoing continuity of care. This thorough documentation protects not only the patient but also you, ensuring a comprehensive record of your professional actions. Accurate and complete records are paramount for legal and ethical reasons, offering a strong defense in any potential legal disputes. Detailed and factual record-keeping is essential for effective practice and protection.

2.3 Shock Treatment

Recognizing shock is paramount; it's not a specific injury but a life-threatening condition. Think of it as your body's desperate cry for help, a cascading failure of its circulatory system. It manifests in various ways, making swift identification crucial. Look for pale, cool, and clammy skin – a classic sign of inadequate blood flow. Rapid, weak pulse, shallow breathing, and altered mental status – from confusion to unconsciousness – are other vital clues. Remember, early detection dramatically improves patient outcomes. Don't just look for one symptom; consider the overall clinical picture.

Hypovolemic shock, the most common type, stems from significant blood or fluid loss. Trauma, internal bleeding, or severe dehydration are frequent culprits. Cardiogenic shock results from the heart's inability to pump blood effectively, often seen in heart attacks. Septic shock arises from overwhelming infection, causing widespread inflammation and circulatory collapse. Neurogenic shock, on the other hand, involves widespread blood vessel dilation, triggered by spinal cord injury or other neurological events. Anaphylactic shock, a severe allergic reaction, also causes a sudden drop in blood pressure. Understanding these different types helps direct your treatment.

Effective management begins with addressing the underlying cause. Control bleeding immediately if that's the problem, using direct pressure, tourniquets, or packing. For cardiogenic shock, supportive measures include oxygen, intravenous fluids, and potentially medication to support heart function. Septic shock requires aggressive fluid resuscitation and antibiotics. In neurogenic shock, careful management of blood pressure, often with medication, is crucial. For anaphylactic shock, administer epinephrine promptly, followed by further support as needed. The key is rapid assessment and targeted intervention, remembering to always check your patient's ABCs: Airway, Breathing, Circulation.

Remember, prompt fluid resuscitation is often vital. Intravenous (IV) fluids replace lost volume and restore blood pressure. The choice and rate of fluid administration depend on the type and severity of shock. Careful monitoring is essential, because giving too much fluid can be as harmful as giving too little. Closely observe the patient's response to treatment, continually assessing vital signs and overall condition. Any change in mental status requires immediate attention. Be aware of potential complications, including acute kidney injury and fluid overload. Precise documentation is vital to ensure continuity of care.

Oxygen administration is another cornerstone of shock management, ensuring adequate tissue oxygenation. High-flow oxygen via a non-rebreather mask is usually the standard. Continuously monitor oxygen saturation levels using pulse oximetry to gauge effectiveness. In severe cases, endotracheal intubation might be necessary to secure the airway and deliver oxygen efficiently. Consider additional airway support for patients with altered mental status or respiratory compromise. Maintaining an open and clear airway is critical throughout the entire process. Your quick thinking and timely intervention could be the difference between life and death for your patient.

Beyond fluid resuscitation and oxygen, consider additional interventions based on the underlying cause. This may involve medications to manage pain, heart rhythm irregularities, or infection. Always remain vigilant for signs of worsening condition, such as decreasing blood pressure or altered mental status. Continuously reassess the patient, adjust treatment as needed, and ensure adequate documentation of all interventions. Regular communication with the emergency medical team is vital to ensure optimal patient care. Teamwork and clear communication are key. Remember to consider the patient's overall condition, and don't hesitate to seek support and advice from senior colleagues. Staying calm and focused is important for your patient and yourself.

Close monitoring is crucial, post-treatment. Vital signs need constant attention, watch for subtle changes that indicate relapse or complications. Regular neurological checks are essential, assessing for any mental status changes, level of consciousness, or focal deficits. Urine output is a valuable indicator of fluid balance and kidney function; low output might signal problems. Be prepared to modify your treatment plan as the patient's condition evolves. Precise, comprehensive documentation is crucial, including the time of intervention, fluids administered, and the patient's response. Continuous monitoring of the patient's condition, even after stabilization, will aid you in providing better care. This diligent follow-up ensures you are always on top of any change in condition.

Remember that treating shock is a dynamic process; your approach will change depending on the patient's response to your interventions. Be prepared to adjust your treatment based on ongoing assessment and observation. Maintain clear communication with your team and the receiving hospital. Effective communication is a lifeline in an emergency setting. Remember that teamwork and careful assessment are critical elements that, combined, make the difference in successfully managing this extremely critical situation. Your professionalism and preparedness are critical assets. Continuous learning and refinement of skills are vital for success in this dynamic field.

3 Chapter 3: Medical Emergencies

Cardiac arrest demands immediate action. Begin chest compressions at a rate of 100-120 per minute, ensuring full chest recoil between compressions. Depth should be at least two inches for adults, adjusting for children and infants. Simultaneously, call for backup and advanced life support, clearly stating the location, patient condition, and actions already taken. Defibrillation, if available, should be administered as soon as possible, following the AED prompts. Intubation and advanced airway management may become necessary depending on the situation and the availability of resources. Remember consistent high-quality CPR is vital until spontaneous circulation returns or definitive care is provided. Maintaining a clear and concise communication log is crucial for post-incident review and legal documentation.

Recognizing a stroke is time-sensitive. Utilize the FAST acronym: Face drooping, Arm weakness, Speech difficulty, Time to call emergency services. Note the exact time of symptom onset; this information is critical for treatment decisions. Assessing the patient's level of consciousness and neurological deficits is essential. Oxygen administration is paramount while awaiting advanced medical support. Precise documentation of symptoms, observations and interventions should be meticulous. Immediate transport to a stroke-capable facility is vital to improve the chances of

effective treatment and minimize long-term disability.
Respiratory distress presents a wide array of causes and severities. Initial assessment should focus on the patient's airway, breathing, and circulation (ABCs). Note respiratory rate, depth, and effort; observe for cyanosis or use of accessory muscles. Administer high-flow oxygen via a non-rebreather mask. Suctioning may be necessary to clear airway secretions. Depending on the severity, consider advanced airway management like bag-valve mask ventilation or endotracheal intubation. Continuous monitoring of vital signs and oxygen saturation is crucial. Remember to document the patient's respiratory pattern, response to interventions, and any changes in their condition.
Seizures require careful observation and management. Protect the patient from injury by removing any nearby hazards. Maintain an open airway and ensure adequate ventilation. Do not restrain the patient unless absolutely necessary to prevent self-harm. Following the seizure, assess the patient's neurological status and vital signs. Document the seizure's duration, characteristics (tonic-clonic, focal, etc.), and the patient's post-ictal state. Consider the possibility of underlying causes and transport the patient to the hospital for further evaluation and treatment. Detailed documentation will provide a comprehensive picture for subsequent medical care.
Anaphylaxis is a life-threatening allergic reaction. Immediate recognition and treatment are crucial. The patient may present with hives, swelling (angioedema), hypotension, and respiratory distress. Administer epinephrine intramuscularly via an auto-injector, following the manufacturer's instructions. Establish and maintain an airway. Administer high-flow oxygen and transport the patient to a hospital. Detailed documentation should include the allergen suspected, timing of symptoms, and the response to treatment. Continuous monitoring of vital signs and ongoing re-assessment are paramount, to guarantee the patient's safe arrival to definitive medical care.

3.1 Cardiac Arrest

Cardiac arrest is a sudden, unexpected loss of heart function. It's a critical emergency requiring immediate intervention. Recognizing the signs—unresponsiveness, absence of breathing or only gasping breaths, and no pulse—is paramount. Time is of the essence; delaying action can have devastating consequences. The chain of survival, a sequence of actions, significantly improves survival chances.

Prompt activation of the emergency response system is the first vital link. A quick call brings trained professionals and equipment to the scene. Early CPR, ideally initiated by a bystander, helps circulate blood and oxygen to the brain and vital organs, buying precious time until advanced life support arrives. Early defibrillation, the use of an automated external defibrillator (AED) to deliver an electric shock to restore a normal heart rhythm, is equally critical. It's a technique that even untrained individuals can master with proper instruction, making AEDs increasingly common in public spaces.

Effective advanced life support (ALS) from paramedics includes administering medications such as epinephrine to stimulate the heart and advanced airway management to ensure sufficient oxygen supply. Intubation, placing a breathing tube into the trachea to assist breathing, is a common procedure in cardiac arrest situations. This ensures a clear airway and allows for efficient oxygen delivery. The paramedic's skill and expertise in these procedures are crucial for the patient's survival.

Intravenous (IV) access is often established to provide medication and fluid support. The placement of an IV line allows for rapid drug administration, bypassing the slower route of intramuscular injection. Careful attention to detail during IV insertion, along with maintaining sterile technique, is important to prevent infection. Once established, the IV line serves as a critical pathway for delivering life-saving interventions.

Continuous monitoring is crucial throughout the resuscitation process. The paramedic must continually assess the patient's response to treatment, adjusting the strategy as needed. This involves monitoring heart rhythm, blood pressure, and oxygen saturation levels, using various monitoring equipment. The interpretation of the collected data guides decisions regarding further interventions. This constant evaluation and adjustment ensure that the most effective approach is used.

Post-cardiac arrest care is equally critical. Once a pulse is restored, the patient isn't out of the woods. They often require intensive care to address the oxygen deprivation their brain and other organs have experienced. Maintaining blood pressure, oxygen levels, and body temperature is paramount in these cases. The paramedic's careful observation of the patient's condition during transport to the hospital contributes significantly to their survival and long-term recovery.

The ability to communicate effectively with the hospital team during the handover process is critical. Clear and concise reporting of the resuscitation events, including interventions, patient response, and medication administered, is essential. This ensures a seamless transition of care, enabling the hospital team to continue life-saving measures promptly and effectively. Using standardized terminology and concise language is crucial during this process.

Effective communication extends beyond the medical team; family members must also be involved. Providing timely updates about the patient's status, providing explanations about what happened, and addressing their concerns with empathy are crucial during this emotional time. This demonstrates professionalism and understanding during an extremely distressing situation. The focus should be on honest, compassionate communication while respecting their emotional state.

Ongoing professional development, through continuing medical education (CME) and regular training, is imperative. Staying updated on the latest guidelines and advancements in cardiac arrest management is crucial for providing the best possible care. This includes hands-on practice to maintain and refine skills, ensuring proficiency in life-saving techniques. The skills and knowledge necessary to manage cardiac arrests effectively constantly evolve. Cardiac arrest is a time-sensitive emergency. Every second counts. The coordinated efforts of bystanders, emergency medical services, and the hospital team can dramatically improve patient outcomes. Proficiency in CPR, the use of AEDs, and advanced life support techniques are crucial elements in achieving this improved outcome. Therefore, continuous learning and the ability to efficiently communicate with multiple stakeholders are paramount in increasing survival rates. A paramedic's proficiency in all these areas saves lives.

3.2 Stroke Recognition

Recognizing a stroke swiftly is paramount. Time is brain, as the saying goes; the faster treatment begins, the better the patient's outcome. Look for the FAST signs: Face drooping, Arm weakness, Speech difficulty, and Time to call emergency services. Don't just focus on one sign; observe the patient holistically. A subtle asymmetry in facial expression, a slight weakness in one arm compared to the other, or slurred speech might be the only indicators initially.

Beyond the FAST acronym, other symptoms often accompany a stroke. These can include sudden numbness or weakness, usually on one side of the body. The patient might experience confusion, trouble seeing in one or both eyes, difficulty with balance and coordination, a severe headache with no known cause, or dizziness. Remember, symptoms vary greatly depending on the location and extent of the brain damage. A thorough assessment requires attentiveness to even minor deviations from normal.

Your initial assessment should be quick but comprehensive. While you're checking vital signs — blood pressure, pulse, and respiratory rate – keep a keen eye on the patient's behavior. Are they alert and oriented? Can they follow simple commands? Are they exhibiting any signs of distress, such as nausea or vomiting? Note the time the symptoms started. Precise timing is crucial for treatment decisions at the hospital. Every second matters in a stroke emergency.

Communication with the patient and their family, if present, is vital. Attempting to communicate with the patient, even if they exhibit speech difficulties, helps in assessing their comprehension and cognitive function. Try simple questions, like "What's your name?" or "Where are you?" Their responses will give you further clues about the severity and nature of the neurological impairment. Reassurance is essential, especially given the frightening nature of the situation.

Document every observation meticulously. Record the time of onset of symptoms, the specific FAST signs observed, and any other relevant symptoms. Note the patient's responses to your questions, their level of consciousness, and any pre-existing medical conditions that could exacerbate the situation. This information will be invaluable to the emergency room physician, aiding in prompt diagnosis and treatment. Clear and concise documentation is crucial for seamless handoff.

Remember the importance of differential diagnosis. Some conditions mimic a stroke, such as hypoglycemia (low blood sugar), seizure, or even migraine headaches. Always consider alternative explanations before reaching a conclusion. However, if you have any suspicion of a stroke, act decisively, as time is of the essence. Do not delay in seeking advanced medical care.

While performing the initial assessment and observing the patient, remember to stay calm and maintain a professional demeanor. Your composure will help reassure the patient and their loved ones. A calm and collected response will ensure you perform the necessary tasks efficiently. This, in turn, will ensure appropriate and timely management of the situation. The patient will appreciate your quiet confidence.

This process of recognition isn't about memorization; it's about understanding the interconnectedness of symptoms. It's about recognizing patterns of neurological deficit. Each case is unique. Don't let your prior experiences blind you to subtle signs. Observe closely, think critically, and act swiftly. This thorough approach will help make a critical difference in outcomes. Your actions, in many cases, will help determine the patient's recovery and future. Never underestimate the importance of teamwork. If you are working in a team, ensure clear communication about your findings and any concerns. A collaborative approach ensures that everyone is informed and working towards the same goal – providing the best possible care to the patient suffering from this emergency condition. The collective expertise can provide a higher degree of confidence and accuracy in diagnosing and managing this life-threatening medical emergency. A united approach is paramount in managing stroke.

Your role extends beyond recognizing a stroke to ensuring efficient and timely transfer to appropriate care. This means coordinating the dispatch of an ambulance and informing the receiving hospital about the patient's condition, time of onset of symptoms, and any initial interventions undertaken. Clear communication is critical in such scenarios, ensuring seamless transitions between care providers. Remember, providing efficient and timely care isn't merely a procedure but a crucial factor that impacts the patient's recovery and overall quality of life. The timely transfer and communication are as vital as the initial recognition.

3.3 Respiratory Distress

Respiratory distress presents a wide spectrum of severity, from mild shortness of breath to life-threatening respiratory failure. Recognizing the subtle differences is paramount. Early identification is crucial, allowing for prompt intervention and potentially preventing a critical situation from escalating. Consider factors like the patient's age, medical history, and the environment; these details significantly influence your assessment. For example, a previously healthy young adult experiencing sudden shortness of breath might require a different approach compared to an elderly patient with chronic obstructive pulmonary disease (COPD) experiencing an exacerbation. This demands a flexible and adaptable approach, requiring you to quickly assess the situation and prioritize your actions.

The initial assessment must be swift and methodical, focusing on the ABCs: airway, breathing, and circulation. Assess the patient's respiratory rate, depth, and effort. Is their breathing shallow and rapid, or deep and labored? Are they using accessory muscles—their neck and shoulder muscles—to breathe? These subtle observations can reveal a lot about the underlying problem. Listen for any unusual sounds like wheezing, rales (crackles), or stridor, each indicative of specific conditions. Wheezing might suggest bronchospasm, while crackles may point towards fluid in the lungs. Stridor, a high-pitched sound, is a sign of upper airway obstruction and requires immediate attention.

Beyond the physical examination, gather a detailed medical history. Previous respiratory issues, allergies, current medications, and recent illnesses all paint a clearer picture. Inquire about any associated symptoms such as chest pain, cough, fever, or changes in mental status. These seemingly minor details can provide vital clues to the cause of the respiratory distress. Remember, a seemingly insignificant cough could signal pneumonia, while chest pain could indicate a pulmonary embolism, a serious condition requiring immediate medical attention. Thorough questioning often provides the missing pieces of the puzzle that guide your clinical decision-making. Efficient questioning requires clear and direct lines of communication, remembering to be both empathetic and professional.

Oxygen therapy is frequently the first-line treatment. Administer supplemental oxygen via a nasal cannula or face mask, aiming for oxygen saturation levels above 94%. Monitoring the patient's response to oxygen is crucial; it indicates whether the underlying problem is primarily hypoxemic or if there's another cause for the distress. In cases of severe respiratory distress, consider high-flow oxygen therapy or non-rebreather masks to deliver a higher concentration of oxygen. Always remember to assess the patient's response continuously to ensure treatment is effective. Continuous monitoring allows you to adjust your approach as needed, ultimately optimizing your treatment strategy.

For patients exhibiting signs of respiratory failure, such as significantly decreased oxygen saturation, altered mental status, or labored breathing, advanced airway management techniques might be necessary. This could involve endotracheal intubation to secure a patent airway and provide mechanical ventilation. However, this procedure requires specialized training and is only to be undertaken by qualified personnel. Remember, incorrect intubation could worsen the patient's condition. Always prioritize your safety and the patient's well-being, working within your scope of practice. Furthermore, this step usually requires teamwork and collaboration with other healthcare professionals, highlighting the importance of clear and concise communication in emergency scenarios.

Beyond immediate interventions, consider potential underlying causes. Conditions ranging from pneumonia and asthma to pulmonary embolism and cardiac failure can manifest as respiratory distress. While a definitive diagnosis is usually made in the hospital setting, your initial assessment and interventions are critical in stabilizing the patient and preventing further deterioration. This requires familiarity with various respiratory conditions and their presentations to anticipate potential needs and rapidly address life-threatening issues. The accuracy of your assessment directly impacts the patient's outcome, emphasizing the importance of continuous learning and skill refinement. Maintaining up-to-date knowledge is crucial for efficient and effective paramedic practice.

Finally, clear communication with the receiving hospital is essential for a seamless transition of care. Concisely relaying your assessment findings, interventions, and the patient's current status is crucial for optimal hospital management. Precise language and accurate terminology avoid ambiguity and ensures the hospital team understands the situation completely. This effective handoff guarantees continuity of care and increases the chances of a successful outcome for the patient. Remember, your role extends beyond the initial response; providing a comprehensive report contributes to the overall success of the treatment plan. Your concise communication is invaluable in ensuring the ongoing care for the patient's needs.

3.4 Seizure Management

Seizures present a unique challenge in prehospital care, demanding rapid assessment and appropriate intervention to protect the patient from harm. The initial priority is always patient safety, focusing on preventing injury during the seizure itself. Protecting the airway is paramount; positioning the patient on their side, into the recovery position, helps to prevent aspiration. We must also clear the immediate area of any objects that could cause further injury during the convulsive episode. Remember to carefully document the entire event, noting the time of onset, duration, and any observed characteristics of the seizure, and the patient's status before, during, and after.

Time is of the essence. The longer the seizure lasts, the greater the risk of complications. Status epilepticus, defined as a seizure lasting longer than five minutes or recurrent seizures without regaining consciousness, represents a life-threatening emergency. Your immediate actions must be decisive and targeted towards mitigating any potential harm while also monitoring the patient's vital signs throughout the entire process. Observe the patient carefully. Noting the duration of the seizure, the body's response, and any post-ictal symptoms is crucial for accurate diagnosis and treatment.

Once the seizure subsides, your focus shifts to post-ictal care. The patient may be drowsy, confused, or disoriented; this is perfectly normal. Maintain a safe environment, monitor vital signs frequently and provide support and reassurance as they regain consciousness, and consider administering oxygen if needed. Be prepared for potential complications like respiratory depression, hypoxia, or cyanosis. Continuous monitoring is necessary until the patient is fully oriented and stable, which should be recorded meticulously.

However, managing a seizure goes beyond immediate crisis management. Gathering a thorough patient history is equally critical. Inquire about the patient's past seizure history, including frequency, duration, precipitating factors, and any prescribed medications. This information provides crucial context, aiding in the determination of the seizure type and severity. Also, any medications the patient is taking must be meticulously accounted for. This is vital for understanding the potential causes and also in preventing unforeseen complications associated with any drug interactions, which can influence your response. This complete history helps make the subsequent treatment more efficient.

Beyond direct seizure management, your role extends to effective communication. Clearly and concisely relaying the patient's condition, the seizure characteristics, and your interventions to the receiving hospital is vital for seamless transfer of care. This information allows the hospital staff to anticipate their needs and prepare for the patient's arrival, enabling a smoother transition into the next stage of care, which also includes accurate documentation for all legal reasons. It is crucial to transmit the vital information to the receiving hospital in a clear, precise, and concise manner so that they can begin preparations to receive the patient.

Remember, your actions must be guided by established protocols and guidelines. Familiarize yourself with local emergency medical service protocols for seizure management. Regularly review and update your knowledge to ensure you're up-to-date on the best practices. Attending continuing medical education courses and engaging in case reviews helps hone your clinical judgement and skills. Always prioritize the patient's safety and well-being above all else. Your calm demeanor, decisive actions, and effective communication are crucial in ensuring a positive outcome.

Effective seizure management requires not only proficiency in immediate interventions but also a comprehensive understanding of the underlying conditions that can cause seizures. This necessitates familiarization with various seizure types, their associated symptoms, and potential causes. Epilepsy, for example, is a common neurological condition that can cause recurrent seizures. Understanding different types of seizures, such as tonic-clonic or absence seizures, is crucial for recognizing the specific need of each patient. Thorough knowledge of these various types can improve the quality of your prehospital care.

Knowing the importance of proper patient care is important, but understanding the legalities involved is equally important. Document every step taken – from initial assessment to hospital handover – with meticulous accuracy. This not only ensures continuity of care but also provides legal protection. Accurate documentation is a crucial element of successful paramedic practice, providing essential clinical evidence and protecting everyone involved. Remember to document all aspects of the episode thoroughly.

Furthermore, continuous learning is essential in this ever-evolving field. Stay abreast of new research, guidelines, and advances in seizure management. Participating in professional development opportunities and staying updated with the latest guidelines is paramount for paramedics. Professional development is necessary to maintain a high standard of care. Your continuing education and professional development enhance your abilities to deliver the best possible patient care, constantly improving your skills and ensuring you remain capable of handling any emergency. The pursuit of knowledge is an ongoing commitment for every paramedic.

Finally, remember that managing seizures is not just a technical skill but also involves empathy and compassion. Patients and their families often experience significant anxiety and fear. Your calm and reassuring presence can provide comfort and support during a stressful and potentially frightening experience. Remember, your role extends beyond medical interventions; it includes providing emotional support. This compassion enhances the healing journey and leaves a positive impact on those in distress.

3.5 Anaphylaxis

Anaphylaxis is a severe, life-threatening allergic reaction. It's crucial to recognize the signs and symptoms rapidly, because early intervention is paramount to preventing death. Time is of the essence; delays can have devastating consequences. Remember, anaphylaxis can progress rapidly, leading to respiratory compromise and cardiovascular collapse within minutes.

The hallmark symptoms of anaphylaxis often include skin manifestations like hives (urticaria), itching, flushing, and angioedema (swelling, particularly around the eyes, lips, and tongue). These skin changes can appear anywhere on the body and are frequently accompanied by respiratory distress. Patients might experience shortness of breath, wheezing, coughing, and even stridor – a high-pitched, whistling sound during breathing that indicates airway narrowing. This is exceptionally serious and needs immediate attention.

Gastrointestinal symptoms are also common, presenting as nausea, vomiting, abdominal cramping, and diarrhea. These symptoms are less reliable indicators of anaphylaxis than the respiratory or cardiovascular signs, however, their presence shouldn't be dismissed. These additional symptoms add to the overall clinical picture, helping in the diagnosis. Remember, the severity of symptoms can vary greatly.

Cardiovascular involvement in anaphylaxis is particularly dangerous. Hypotension (low blood pressure) can occur rapidly, leading to shock and potentially cardiac arrest. Tachycardia (rapid heart rate) is another frequent finding and signifies the body's struggle to compensate for the effects of the allergic reaction. These cardiovascular signs are typically later in the presentation than skin or respiratory symptoms but are very significant and indicate the need for prompt treatment. This is why early recognition is so critical.

Your initial assessment should focus on securing the airway and supporting breathing. If the patient is having trouble breathing, administer high-flow oxygen immediately. This immediate intervention is often life-saving in the setting of anaphylactic shock. If the patient is unconscious or showing signs of respiratory failure, intubation or bag-valve-mask ventilation might be necessary. Always maintain a patent airway while you manage other aspects of care.

Epinephrine (adrenaline) is the cornerstone of anaphylaxis treatment. It's crucial to administer it intramuscularly into the outer thigh; this is the most effective and rapid route for absorption and the best way to reverse the effects quickly. The dose depends on the patient's age and weight, so follow established protocols precisely. It is essential to document what medication, and the dose was administered. Remember, time is a critical factor in anaphylactic shock, so prompt administration of epinephrine is not only recommended but essential.

Supporting circulation is just as important as managing the airway. This often involves intravenous fluid resuscitation, using crystalloid solutions like normal saline or Ringer's lactate to improve blood pressure and tissue perfusion. Monitor the patient's blood pressure frequently; this will give you a clear indication of the effectiveness of the fluid resuscitation efforts. This also helps to show the impact of administered drugs. Closely monitor hemodynamics.

After administering epinephrine and providing supportive care, the patient requires ongoing monitoring for any recurrence of symptoms. Many patients can experience a biphasic reaction, meaning symptoms can reappear hours after the initial episode. Therefore, even if the patient seems to have recovered fully, you must monitor them for a significant period post-administration of epinephrine. This is a critical safety step, especially in life threatening conditions.

The patient requires immediate transport to a hospital for further evaluation and management. Continuous monitoring of vital signs, respiratory status, and cardiac rhythm is necessary throughout the transport phase. Close monitoring should continue even in the hospital setting. Close communication with the receiving hospital is also crucial to ensure the patient receives appropriate ongoing care. It's important to provide a thorough handover report to the emergency department physician, detailing the assessment, treatment, and response. This smooth transition of care is crucial for a good outcome.

Remember, anaphylaxis is a medical emergency. Your prompt and skillful intervention can make a life-or-death difference. Accurate communication with your team, precise documentation, and careful adherence to established protocols are paramount. Your role as a paramedic is to act quickly, decisively, and competently, working efficiently as a team. Efficient and calm teamwork is of the highest importance, as well as good communication with the patient and family, building rapport with them and explaining what you are doing. Never underestimate the importance of clear communication and proper documentation in all medical emergency situations.

4 Chapter 4: Pediatric Cases

The airway in infants and young children differs significantly from that of adults. Their tongues are proportionally larger, their airways are narrower, and their tracheas are more flexible. This means that even a slight obstruction can quickly lead to respiratory compromise. During CPR, proper head positioning is paramount to prevent airway blockage. The chin lift maneuver, while effective in adults, may be insufficient in infants, potentially causing spinal cord injury. Instead, the jaw thrust maneuver is preferred. Remember, maintaining a patent airway is the absolute priority. Failure to do so can rapidly lead to irreversible brain damage due to hypoxia, highlighting the critical need for immediate and skillful intervention.

Assessing a child requires a different approach than assessing an adult. You can't simply ask a toddler what hurts; their communication skills are limited, and relying solely on their verbal responses would be insufficient and potentially inaccurate. Therefore, you must observe their behavior, posture and interactions, noting their overall demeanor. A quiet, withdrawn child might indicate pain or illness, whereas an excessively irritable child might suggest discomfort, infection, or other underlying conditions. Gathering information from parents or caregivers is essential; they often provide valuable insights into the child's medical history, allergies,

and typical behavior. This comprehensive assessment, combining observation with parental input, is crucial for identifying the underlying issue and formulating an appropriate treatment plan.
Infant CPR differs significantly from adult CPR. The compression-to-ventilation ratio is different, and the depth and rate of compressions are adjusted based on the infant's size and age. Two fingers, rather than the heel of the hand, are used for chest compressions. The correct hand placement is crucial to avoid injury to the delicate ribs and underlying organs. Furthermore, the technique itself requires a more gentle approach, given the infant's smaller and more fragile chest cavity. The rescuer must ensure that the compressions are effective but not forceful enough to cause harm. This gentler approach makes it more effective for the rescuer to keep good circulation and to avoid fatigue during the process.
Recognizing the signs and symptoms of various conditions in children can be challenging due to their developmental stage. A fever, for example, might manifest differently in a toddler than in a teenager. A young child may exhibit lethargy and irritability, while an older child may exhibit more classic symptoms like headache and muscle aches. Similarly, respiratory distress in infants might present as grunting or nasal flaring, whereas in older children, it may present as increased respiratory rate and shortness of breath. Understanding the age-appropriate presentation of various conditions is critical for a prompt and accurate diagnosis. Learning to correctly interpret those changes is imperative to provide adequate treatment and care.
Proper documentation of pediatric cases is crucial. It must include not only vital signs and treatment administered but also observations of the child's behavior, parent interactions, and response to treatment. Including details such as the child's developmental stage, any pre-existing medical conditions, and the response of the child's physical environment are critical elements. This detailed approach ensures the provision of quality care and also protects the paramedic and the child, in case of legal issues or for future reference. Incomplete or inaccurate documentation

can have serious legal and ethical consequences, and could lead to inadequate follow-up care. Thorough documentation protects both the child and the practitioner.

Dealing with anxious parents during a pediatric emergency requires patience and empathy. Parents often experience intense fear and helplessness when their child is ill or injured. Your role is not just to treat the child but to also reassure the parents and keep them informed. Open and honest communication, explaining the steps being taken and the child's condition in simple terms, can help to ease their anxiety. Remember, creating a supportive atmosphere is vital for both the child and the parents. This approach requires a sensitivity to their emotional states and a willingness to share information honestly. This builds a positive doctor-patient relationship. This calm and sensitive approach can significantly impact the overall emergency response.

Dealing with a pediatric trauma case requires a modified approach. While the principles of trauma management remain the same, the specific techniques need adaptation to account for the child's smaller size and developing physiology. For instance, splinting a child's fracture requires smaller, more flexible splints than those used for adults. Bleeding control in infants and young children often involves different techniques because their blood volume is much lower than an adult. These are crucial details that can have a drastic impact on the success of the treatment. Even small differences in technique can affect the outcome in these very small patients.

Age-appropriate communication is critical in providing the best possible care to pediatric patients. Speaking directly to the child, adapting your language to their developmental level and age, fosters trust and cooperation. Explaining procedures in simple terms and offering choices, when appropriate, can minimize fear and anxiety. Remember, children respond to your tone and demeanor. Being calm and gentle can ease their distress. A playful and reassuring approach makes the overall experience easier on the child. A calm voice can help to keep the child calm, especially if the child

is younger.
When transporting a pediatric patient, maintaining appropriate thermoregulation is crucial. Infants and young children are highly susceptible to hypothermia and hyperthermia. Proper use of blankets, warming devices, or cooling measures during transportation is essential to prevent adverse outcomes. Monitoring the child's temperature and providing supplemental warmth or cooling as needed is crucial throughout the transport process. This will minimize the risks and assure the best possible care for the patient. These adjustments are also crucial for the well-being of the child during transport, even during mild weather conditions.
In summary, pediatric emergency care requires specialized knowledge and skills. Understanding the unique physiological differences between children and adults is paramount for providing effective care. By mastering the specific techniques for airway management, CPR, assessment, communication, and transport, paramedics can significantly improve the outcomes for these vulnerable patients. Remember, a comprehensive and patient-centered approach is key to successfully managing pediatric emergency situations. This holistic approach guarantees that the children receive the best possible care, while maintaining the safety of the child.

4.1 Infant CPR

Infant CPR differs significantly from adult CPR, demanding a nuanced approach. Remember, swift action is paramount, as infants' small size and delicate anatomy necessitate gentler yet equally effective techniques. Time is critical in these situations; every second counts.
The first step involves checking for responsiveness. Gently tap the infant's feet and shout, "Are you okay?". Absence of response necessitates immediate action. If you find no response, immediately

call for emergency medical services. Simultaneously, begin CPR. Next, open the airway. Use the head-tilt-chin-lift maneuver, but with gentler pressure than you would use on an adult to avoid injuring the infant's neck. Ensure the infant's head is not overextended or flexed too much. Check for breathing. Look, listen, and feel for normal breathing for no more than 10 seconds. The absence of normal breathing or only gasping breaths triggers the commencement of chest compressions.

Chest compressions are crucial. Two fingers should be placed on the breastbone, just below the nipple line. Compress the chest at a rate of 100 to 120 compressions per minute, to a depth of about one-and-a-half inches. Allow the chest to fully recoil after each compression. Continuous compressions are vital; pausing can be detrimental.

After 30 chest compressions, deliver two rescue breaths. Seal the infant's mouth and nose completely with your mouth, creating an airtight seal. Give two slow breaths, each lasting about one second, and watch for chest rise. If the chest does not rise, re-position the airway and try again before resuming compressions.

The cycle of 30 compressions and two breaths continues until help arrives or the infant begins to breathe normally. It's essential to maintain a consistent rhythm and depth of compressions throughout the procedure. Avoid interruptions unless absolutely necessary. Fatigue is a real concern, so consider switching rescuers if possible.

Remember, infant CPR is a demanding procedure. Regular training and practice are essential to ensure proficiency. The knowledge gained from this course should not replace professional training; it's a crucial addition to your skillset. Certification courses provide hands-on experience and reinforce critical techniques.

While performing CPR, maintaining a clear communication channel with the emergency medical services is vital. Providing them with accurate information about the infant's condition and your actions enables them to prepare appropriately before arrival. Ac-

curate reporting is as vital as the CPR itself.
Effective communication during the crisis is paramount. Use clear and concise language, relaying essential information to the emergency responders. A calm and organized approach is crucial for both the infant's well-being and your own composure.
Following the emergency, post-incident documentation is essential. Recording details of the incident, including your actions and the infant's response, aids in subsequent medical care and serves as crucial evidence for any legal or investigative purposes. Precise record-keeping is critical for professional liability.
Finally, remember the importance of emotional support. Providing infant CPR is emotionally challenging. Seeking support from colleagues or supervisors following a difficult situation is crucial for both your personal well-being and professional resilience. Accessing debriefing sessions can aid in processing the experience. It is vital to address the mental health aspects of this profession. Your own well-being is just as important as the well-being of your patients.

4.2 Child Assessment

Assessing a child differs significantly from assessing an adult. Their smaller size, less developed communication skills, and rapidly changing physiological parameters require a modified approach. Remember, a calm and reassuring demeanor is paramount; a frightened child will not cooperate easily, hindering your assessment. Your first priority is always to ensure the child's safety and comfort. Begin by establishing a rapport with the child and their parent or guardian if possible. A gentle smile and a soft voice go a long way.
Observe the child from a distance before approaching. Note their overall appearance, level of alertness, and respiratory effort. Are they crying inconsolably? Do they seem lethargic or unresponsive? These initial observations can provide vital clues to their

condition. Take note of their position—are they curled up in pain, or are they lying limply? Any unusual positioning could indicate injury or discomfort. Always prioritize a systematic approach, beginning with the ABCs: airway, breathing, and circulation. Assess the airway for any obstructions, breathing for rate, rhythm, and depth, and circulation for pulse and capillary refill.

While obtaining vital signs, remember age-appropriate techniques. For example, use a smaller blood pressure cuff to ensure accurate readings. Counting the respiratory rate can be done by observing the chest rise and fall. Consider the child's developmental stage; a toddler's responses will differ from a teenager's. Always involve the parents or guardians in the process if they are present and willing to participate, because their knowledge of the child's medical history, allergies, and typical behaviour is invaluable. Try to ascertain the history of the present illness from the parents. When was the child last well? What symptoms prompted them to seek medical attention? These details are essential for accurate diagnosis and treatment.

Pay close attention to the child's response to your touch. Are they flinching in pain? Do they react to stimuli? Check for any obvious injuries like cuts, bruises, or deformities. Remember that children may not be able to articulate their pain accurately; instead, they may express it through crying, irritability, or changes in behavior. Observe the child's skin; is it pale, flushed, or mottled? These subtle changes can indicate significant underlying problems. Assess the child's hydration status; are their mucous membranes dry? Are their eyes sunken? These observations help determine the severity of dehydration, a common issue in children.

Remember the pediatric assessment triangle: appearance, work of breathing, and circulation to the skin. These three components provide a quick overview of the child's condition. A child with altered mental status, significant respiratory distress, or poor perfusion is in critical condition and requires immediate intervention. While performing the physical exam, use age-appropriate communication techniques. Explain what you are doing in simple terms. Distraction techniques, such as talking about toys or games, can help keep the child calm and cooperative. Remember, documentation is crucial; accurately record all findings, including vital signs, observations, and interventions. Thorough documentation helps ensure continuity of care and protects both the child and the paramedic.

Finally, always be aware of the emotional needs of both the child and their parents. A stressful situation can be overwhelming for everyone involved. Providing reassurance and support can significantly improve the outcome. Remember, effective communication and a patient-centered approach are just as important as the technical aspects of assessment. Your calm demeanor and ability to build rapport are essential tools for successful pediatric care. The ability to quickly and accurately assess a child is crucial in emergency situations, potentially saving their life. Never underestimate the value of a calm, reassuring presence, and always remember the child's age and developmental stage as you conduct your assessment. Thorough and careful assessments lead to accurate diagnoses and treatment plans, improving the chance of positive outcomes for young patients. This comprehensive approach will contribute to effective care and ultimately, better patient outcomes.

5 Chapter 5: Geriatric Patients

Geriatric patients present unique challenges for paramedics. Their physiology differs significantly from younger adults, requiring a modified approach to assessment and treatment. Understanding these differences is paramount to providing safe and effective care. For instance, consider that even a seemingly minor fall can result in serious injury due to decreased bone density and muscle mass, a common occurrence often leading to hip fractures and other complications. Accurate assessment and prompt intervention are crucial to minimize long-term consequences.

Falls are frequent occurrences among elderly individuals, often resulting from a combination of factors including decreased balance, muscle weakness, medication side effects, and environmental hazards. Assessing the fall itself is as important as assessing the patient's injuries. Consider the circumstances surrounding the fall—was it a simple stumble, or did a medical event contribute to the fall? This understanding influences treatment and can potentially prevent future falls. Document the details thoroughly, noting any pre-existing conditions or medications that may have played a role.

Medication reconciliation is critically important in geriatric patients, many of whom are on multiple medications (polypharmacy). This practice involves comparing the patient's current medication list with their medical records, as well as any new prescriptions or over-the-counter drugs they might be taking. Discrepancies and potential adverse drug interactions can be identified, potentially preventing serious complications. Always ask the patient, their family, or their caregiver about the exact medications they're currently taking, including dosages and timing. It's crucial to look for potential interactions. For example, the combined use of certain blood thinners and antiplatelet agents can greatly increase bleeding risks.

Polypharmacy, the concurrent use of multiple medications, significantly increases the risk of adverse drug reactions in geriatric patients. These reactions can manifest in various ways, ranging from mild side effects like dizziness and nausea to life-threatening complications such as bleeding, heart problems, or falls. Understanding the potential interactions between different medications is crucial for paramedics, as such interactions can severely compromise the patient's health. When dealing with a geriatric patient exhibiting confusion, disorientation, or unusual symptoms, review their medication list for any known interactions. This knowledge can be lifesaving.

Another key aspect of geriatric care is recognizing the altered presentation of common medical conditions. For example, symptoms of heart attack or stroke might be atypical in elderly patients. They may not experience the classic crushing chest pain associated with a heart attack, instead presenting with shortness of breath, fatigue, or nausea. Similarly, the signs of stroke might be subtle and easily overlooked, such as mild weakness or confusion. Therefore, maintaining a high index of suspicion for these conditions and performing a thorough assessment is vital, paying close attention to any subtle changes or seemingly unrelated symptoms.

Assessing the mental status of an elderly patient is also essential. Confusion, disorientation, or changes in behavior can be indicative of underlying medical issues, such as infections, dehydration, medication side effects, or even a stroke. Using a standardized assessment tool can help ensure consistency and completeness. Be aware of the patient's baseline cognitive function—if possible, try to obtain information from family members or caregivers about any recent cognitive changes. This context is crucial in differentiating between normal age-related changes and potentially serious conditions.

Communication with geriatric patients and their families requires patience and sensitivity. Many elderly patients have impaired hearing or vision, affecting communication. Speak clearly and slowly, maintaining good eye contact. Use simple language, avoiding medical jargon. Always ensure that the patient, or their legally appointed representative, understands the information provided and gives informed consent before any treatment is given. Family involvement can be invaluable, providing crucial information about the patient's medical history and preferences.

Finally, remember that geriatric patients are individuals. Avoid generalizations. Every patient's situation is unique, influenced by their medical history, current condition, and personal circumstances. Thorough assessment, careful medication reconciliation, awareness of polypharmacy risks, and excellent communication skills are integral components of providing the best possible care to this vulnerable population. Treat each case as a unique puzzle, piecing together information to create the most appropriate intervention plan. Remember your role is vital in ensuring their safety and well-being.

5.1 Fall Management

Falls are a significant concern for geriatric patients, often leading to serious injuries and decreased quality of life. Understanding the multifaceted nature of fall management requires a systematic approach encompassing pre-fall risk assessment, intervention strategies, and post-fall care. This involves not just treating the immediate injuries but also identifying and addressing underlying contributing factors. Effective communication with the patient, their family, and other healthcare professionals is paramount throughout this process.

Assessing fall risk involves a thorough review of the patient's medical history, including medication regimen, cognitive status, mobility limitations, visual acuity, and environmental factors within their home. For instance, a history of syncope or orthostatic hypotension significantly increases fall risk, while medications like sedatives or antihypertensives can exacerbate the problem. Visual impairments and reduced mobility due to arthritis or other conditions are further risk factors demanding attention. Similarly, poorly lit hallways or tripping hazards at home contribute significantly to fall probability. A detailed history provides the necessary context for personalized intervention. Remember to always document your findings meticulously for future reference and continuity of care. Clear and concise documentation is essential for successful communication and care planning.

Interventions aimed at preventing falls are highly individualized and depend upon the patient's specific risk profile. These can range from simple measures like improving home lighting and removing obstacles, to more complex interventions such as physical therapy programs to improve strength, balance, and gait. In some cases, assistive devices, like walkers or canes, might be necessary, while others might benefit from medication adjustments to minimize side effects that increase fall risk. Regular review of medication lists is crucial, working collaboratively with the patient's physician to assess the necessity and potential risks of each medication. This process, often referred to as medication reconciliation, ensures that the patient's medication regimen is safe and effective, minimizing the chances of adverse interactions that might impair balance or cognition.

Following a fall, immediate assessment of injuries is crucial, employing the standard protocols for trauma assessment. This prioritizes identification and management of life-threatening conditions like head injuries, spinal fractures, and internal bleeding. After stabilizing the patient's condition, comprehensive assessment focuses on identifying the cause of the fall, assessing for underlying medical issues that might have contributed, and evaluating the severity of any injuries. This requires careful observation of the patient's physical and cognitive state, and this should ideally involve discussions with the patient, family members, or caretakers if appropriate and possible to gather information regarding the circumstances of the fall.

Post-fall management extends beyond treating immediate injuries; it addresses the underlying vulnerabilities that increased the risk. This often involves a multidisciplinary approach, involving geriatricians, physical therapists, occupational therapists, and social workers. Physical therapy plays a vital role in restoring mobility and balance, while occupational therapy addresses adaptive strategies for managing daily activities to reduce future fall risk. Social workers can assess and address environmental factors within the patient's home or other social determinants impacting their safety and independence. It may also involve adjustments to the patient's home environment or the implementation of support services to help them remain safe and independent. This integrated approach aims not only to treat the immediate consequences of the fall but also to reduce the likelihood of future falls, thereby improving the patient's quality of life and reducing the burden on the healthcare system. The holistic approach is key to improving outcomes and emphasizing the importance of teamwork across disciplines. Your role as a paramedic is to initiate this process with accurate assessment, timely intervention and seamless transition to other healthcare providers. You are a critical link in this collaborative effort.

5.2 Medication Reconciliation

Medication reconciliation is a critical, often overlooked, step in providing safe and effective care to geriatric patients. It involves comparing the patient's current medication list with their home medication list and any other recent medication records. This process helps identify discrepancies and potential interactions that could lead to adverse events, particularly in elderly individuals who frequently take multiple medications. Failing to perform this crucial step can result in medication errors that have severe consequences, including hospital readmissions and increased mortality. Therefore, thoroughness is paramount.

The elderly population often suffers from multiple chronic conditions requiring simultaneous medications. This "polypharmacy" increases the risk of drug interactions, both synergistic and antagonistic. Some medications can exacerbate underlying health issues, while others might interact negatively, leading to unexpected side effects or reduced therapeutic efficacy. A careful comparison of medication lists, therefore, doesn't just identify missing or duplicate prescriptions; it also highlights potential conflicts that need immediate attention. Consider, for example, the potential interaction between a blood thinner and an antiplatelet agent. Such a combination might greatly increase the risk of bleeding.

To perform effective medication reconciliation, begin by obtaining a complete list of the patient's current medications. This should include prescription drugs, over-the-counter medications, herbal supplements, and even vitamins. Ask the patient, their family members, or caregivers for this information. Review any available medication bottles, packaging, or other documentation. Remember to include dosage, frequency, and the last time the medication was taken. Sometimes, patients might be unaware of all the medications they're currently using, or might have difficulty recalling details due to cognitive impairment, so careful questioning and a thorough search for information are critical.

Next, obtain a list of the medications the patient typically takes at home. This could come from the patient's own records, their pharmacy, or their physician. This step is crucial because it provides a baseline for comparison. Discrepancies between the home medication list and the current medication list are highlighted, indicating possible errors or omissions. A missing medication might indicate a need for continuation, while an extra medication might reveal an accidental duplicate prescription or an unintentional overdose. Compare both lists item by item, carefully noting any differences.

Once you have both lists, meticulously compare them. Look for any discrepancies, such as missing medications, extra medications, dosage changes, or changes in frequency. Consider also any known drug interactions that might be present. This requires a good understanding of pharmacology and the potential interactions between various medications. Utilize readily available online resources or consult a pharmacist if needed for clarification. This thorough check ensures you catch potentially hazardous situations early.

After identifying discrepancies, document all findings clearly and concisely in the patient's medical record. This documentation serves as a legal record of the medication reconciliation process. It ensures accountability and allows for continuous monitoring. Remember to report any significant findings to the patient's physician or other appropriate healthcare provider. These reported discrepancies need timely resolution, to prevent potential adverse effects on the patient.

Finally, remember that effective medication reconciliation requires communication and collaboration. Communicate clearly and concisely with patients, family members, and other healthcare professionals. Work together to ensure the patient receives the correct medications in the right dosages. This collaborative approach ensures patient safety and improves the overall quality of care. Clear communication prevents misunderstandings and helps resolve any discrepancies swiftly. The end goal is not just to identify discrepancies, but to actively resolve them and ensure the patient's safe transition to a continuing care plan or discharge. This attention to detail can significantly improve the outcome of treatment and reduce potential risks.

Medication reconciliation isn't just a task; it's a crucial aspect of ensuring patient safety, especially for our geriatric patients. It's a testament to our commitment to providing the best possible care. The meticulous process demands attention to detail, teamwork, and a thorough understanding of pharmacology, ultimately contributing to better patient outcomes and preventing potentially life-threatening errors. Remember this: attention to detail, thorough record-keeping, and effective communication are the cornerstones of successful medication reconciliation.

5.3 Polypharmacy Considerations

Geriatric patients often take multiple medications, a practice known as polypharmacy. This presents unique challenges for paramedics, demanding a keen awareness of potential drug interactions and their impact on patient presentation. Understanding the complexities of polypharmacy is crucial for safe and effective care. Failure to recognize the cumulative effects of multiple medications can lead to misdiagnosis, inappropriate treatment, and potentially dangerous outcomes.

Recognizing polypharmacy begins with a thorough medication reconciliation. This involves meticulously reviewing all the patient's medications, including prescription drugs, over-the-counter remedies, and herbal supplements. This isn't simply listing the medications; it's actively seeking information about dosages, frequency, and the reason for each prescription. Engage the patient, their family, or their caregivers – anyone who can offer a clear and complete picture of their medication regime. Don't hesitate to ask detailed questions; clarifying information can be the key to accurate assessment.

The information gathered during medication reconciliation is invaluable. It lays the groundwork for recognizing potential drug interactions. Some interactions are synergistic, enhancing the effects of individual drugs, while others are antagonistic, potentially counteracting the intended effects. Certain medications can also exacerbate underlying conditions or cause entirely new symptoms, masking the actual medical emergency. For example, a patient presenting with confusion might be experiencing a side effect of multiple medications, rather than a stroke or other neurological event. Thorough record-keeping is essential, both to prevent errors and to facilitate collaboration with other healthcare providers involved in the patient's care.

Be aware that certain medications frequently associated with polypharmacy, such as anticoagulants, antiplatelet agents, and sedatives, can significantly alter a patient's presentation and response to treatment. Anticoagulants increase the risk of bleeding, requiring extra caution during procedures or even simply handling the patient. Similarly, sedatives can mask symptoms of various conditions, potentially delaying appropriate interventions. Antiplatelet agents increase the risk of bruising, which can be confused with traumatic injuries. Understanding the potential effects of these medications will guide your assessment and treatment decisions, preventing potential complications.

The consequences of failing to account for polypharmacy can be severe. Adverse drug reactions are a common complication of polypharmacy, ranging from mild side effects to life-threatening events. These reactions can manifest in diverse ways, mimicking the symptoms of other medical emergencies. This could result in misdiagnosis and inappropriate treatment, potentially worsening the patient's condition. Accurate medication information, coupled with a thorough understanding of potential drug interactions, is crucial for making informed decisions and providing the best possible care. Consult relevant resources if unsure, and never hesitate to seek additional medical guidance when needed.

Furthermore, the impact of polypharmacy extends beyond immediate treatment decisions. Careful documentation of the patient's medication regimen, along with your assessment of potential interactions and their impact on the patient's condition, is essential for continuity of care. This comprehensive documentation enables effective communication with other healthcare providers involved in the patient's treatment, improving the overall quality of care and minimizing the risk of medication errors or adverse events. Moreover, this detailed recording provides vital information for future medical encounters, helping to prevent similar complications in the future.

Beyond medication interactions, consider the cognitive impact of polypharmacy. Many medications used by elderly patients, particularly those with multiple comorbidities, can affect cognitive function. Confusion, disorientation, and memory problems are common side effects. These effects can confound the assessment process, making it harder to obtain an accurate history and establish the patient's baseline mental state. Understanding these potential cognitive changes is essential for adapting communication strategies and eliciting necessary information effectively and efficiently. Clear communication strategies are essential, including asking simple questions and providing clear, concise instructions to minimize the likelihood of misunderstandings caused by altered cognitive function.

In conclusion, managing geriatric patients effectively requires an understanding of polypharmacy's complex challenges. Medication reconciliation is the cornerstone of safe care, providing a comprehensive overview of the patient's medication profile. Recognition of potential drug interactions is crucial for avoiding misdiagnosis and preventing adverse outcomes. Don't underestimate the cognitive impact of multiple medications; adapting your communication style is essential for efficient assessment and effective patient care. Thorough documentation safeguards continuity of care and contributes to improved patient outcomes. By actively addressing polypharmacy, paramedics can ensure the best possible care for their geriatric patients.

6 Chapter 6: Reporting & Documentation

Precise and timely documentation is paramount in emergency medical services. Your reports aren't just records; they're legal shields, vital pieces of a patient's medical journey, and crucial learning tools for future interventions. Every detail matters, from the initial call to the hospital handover.

Incident reports demand accuracy. Begin by clearly stating the date, time, and location of the incident. Record the nature of the call, including the dispatcher's information and the initial complaint. Detail every action you took, from your arrival to the patient's transfer to the receiving facility. List the equipment used, and note any challenges encountered. Objectively describe the scene, the patient's condition, and the interventions employed. Don't forget to document the patient's response to your treatment, whether it was positive, negative, or neutral. Thoroughness safeguards you and ensures consistent high-quality care. Leave no stone unturned; every seemingly minor detail contributes to the complete picture.

Patient charts serve as the ongoing record of a patient's care. They should be comprehensive, clear, and concise, adhering strictly to the established medical charting standards and your organization's protocols. Include all vital signs, medications administered, and treatments provided, always specifying the time each action occurred. Document the patient's response to treatments, detailing observed changes in their condition. Use precise medical terminology, avoiding colloquialisms or subjective assessments. If you face any ethical dilemmas or challenges in a particular case, meticulously document the conflict, how you addressed it, and the decision made. Note also any patient refusals, making sure that the reasons for refusal and any attempts at persuasion are adequately detailed. Accuracy in recording these details protects both the paramedic and the patient and can be beneficial if legal issues arise.

Remember, your documentation protects you. Inaccuracies or omissions can jeopardize your reputation and even lead to legal repercussions. Clear, concise, and objective reporting not only satisfies legal requirements but also facilitates efficient communication and ensures continuity of care. Consistently maintaining high standards of reporting fosters a culture of accountability and continuous improvement within the emergency medical services. Always utilize approved abbreviations and never use jargon, to ensure everyone easily understands your notes.

Consider using a structured approach to recording your findings. Employing a standardized reporting format minimizes the risk of omissions and ensures all critical information is consistently documented. This organized style helps other medical professionals quickly understand the patient's history and the course of treatment. Furthermore, a methodical and well-structured approach simplifies later review and minimizes potential misunderstandings.

Beyond the immediate needs of the patient and your own protection, accurate reporting is a valuable resource for future care. Your thorough documentation serves as a detailed account of the situation, providing invaluable information for research and improving emergency medical practices. Well-documented cases can significantly contribute to medical knowledge, helping to refine treatment protocols and enhance patient outcomes in the future.

Never underestimate the significance of detailed documentation.

It's not just about fulfilling administrative duties; it's about upholding your professional responsibilities. Your notes serve as a comprehensive account of the patient's experience, which could be crucial for further treatment or legal processes. The clear and concise nature of your writing protects both the patient and yourself, making it indispensable in the field of emergency medicine. Always double check your work for clarity, accuracy and completeness. Make sure that your notes provide a clear and easily understandable picture of the situation.

Effective documentation isn't merely a series of facts; it's a narrative of a critical moment in a patient's life. Every detail, meticulously recorded, paints a richer picture of their medical history, treatment, and response. This narrative contributes not only to the immediate needs of the patient but also to the collective body of medical knowledge, helping shape and improve future practices and enhancing safety standards.

In conclusion, proficient reporting and documentation are not merely administrative tasks; they are fundamental to ensuring safe, effective, and ethical practice in emergency medical services. Precise, detailed, and objective documentation safeguards both patients and paramedics, forms the basis for continuous improvement, and contributes to the advancement of medical knowledge. Make it a habit, and make it a priority.

6.1 Incident Reports

Accurate and complete incident reports are crucial for several reasons. They serve as a vital record of the events surrounding an emergency call, protecting both the patient and the paramedic team. This documentation is essential for improving future responses and ensuring accountability. Negligence in reporting can lead to serious consequences, including legal repercussions and damage to professional reputation. Therefore, meticulous attention to detail is paramount.

A well-written incident report begins with the basic information: date, time, location, and the names of all personnel involved. This foundational information provides an immediate context for the events described later in the report. Next, the report should meticulously detail the circumstances leading to the emergency call. This could include the nature of the call, the dispatch information received, and any preliminary information gleaned from bystanders or witnesses. The accuracy of this section is critical, as any discrepancies could impact the overall narrative. Remember to include the exact time the unit was dispatched and the exact time the unit arrived on the scene. These precise time stamps are essential when analyzing response times. You should also include any difficulties faced during the response like traffic conditions and accessibility challenges, noting any delays incurred and their reasons. Always be objective; emotions and personal opinions have no place in a formal report.

The patient assessment section of the report requires a comprehensive and systematic approach. Document the patient's vital signs—heart rate, blood pressure, respiratory rate, temperature, and oxygen saturation—clearly and precisely. The chief complaint should be clearly stated, followed by a detailed account of the patient's symptoms and medical history. Record any allergies or current medications the patient is taking. If there are pre-existing conditions, those must be explicitly included. It is crucial that any observations are recorded objectively, without personal interpretation or subjective feelings. This section forms the core of the medical evidence contained within the report and should be treated as such. The information given by the patient should be recorded faithfully without adding any analysis of the information.

Moving beyond initial assessment, the interventions performed by your team should be precisely outlined in a chronological order. Describe each procedure in detail, including the specific equipment used, dosages of medications administered, and the patient's response to each intervention. Any complications encountered during treatment should also be documented, alongside the steps taken to mitigate them. For example, if intravenous access proved difficult, that should be stated, including the number of attempts made and the reason for any challenges. Documenting the rationale behind decisions, including why certain treatment paths were chosen, demonstrates thorough consideration and professional judgment.

The report should conclude with the patient's condition upon transfer or discharge, including where they were transferred to and the method of transfer – ambulance, helicopter or other means of transport. You need to specify the condition in which the patient was left, including relevant notes about any ongoing care needed. After the patient's condition, you need to include the time you handed over your patient to another healthcare provider. For example, when you left a patient to the care of the emergency room physician. The entire report should adhere to the established guidelines and formats of your employing agency. Inconsistencies or omissions can impact the legal validity of the document and potentially hinder any subsequent investigations or legal proceedings. The process and outcome of the call need to be thoroughly explained and analyzed to allow for future learning and prevent similar incidents. Therefore, take the time and follow the reporting protocol properly.

Finally, remember that the incident report is not just a piece of paperwork; it's a vital tool for learning, improving, and safeguarding both your professional practice and the well-being of future patients. By diligently completing these reports, you contribute to a safer and more effective emergency medical system. Take your time and document everything thoroughly. Always double check your work before filing. Remember, accuracy and completeness are paramount.

6.2 Patient Charts

Patient charts are the cornerstone of effective paramedic practice, serving as a crucial record of the patient's journey from initial assessment to final disposition. They're not merely administrative tasks; they're legal documents, vital for continuity of care, and a powerful tool in ensuring the safety and wellbeing of your patients. Maintaining meticulously accurate and complete charts is paramount, and the details you record will directly impact future medical decisions. Therefore, understanding the key components and best practices is essential.

The information you record must adhere to stringent standards, encompassing a comprehensive range of data points. From the moment you first encounter the patient, each observation, procedure, and medication administered must be documented clearly and concisely, following established protocols within your organization. Failure to do so can lead to legal ramifications, hindering effective treatment and potentially endangering patients. Therefore, accuracy is not just desirable; it is mandatory.

Your chart should provide a clear narrative, painting a vivid picture of the events unfolding during the emergency. It shouldn't just list facts; it should tell a story, albeit a concise one. Start by clearly stating the time of your arrival and the initial scene assessment—Was the scene safe? Were there any bystanders? Detailed descriptions are necessary, allowing for a thorough reconstruction of the incident should it ever be needed. Your notes need to make sense to anyone looking at them, not just you.

Consider including specific details about the patient's presentation, including physical findings. These objective findings provide crucial context that complements subjective details. Was the patient conscious and alert, or unresponsive? Note the patient's vital signs – heart rate, blood pressure, respiratory rate, oxygen saturation, and temperature – and record them at regular intervals, showing the trend of change. It's essential to note the presence of any abnormalities, such as abnormal skin colour, or unusual smells, because they might point to underlying conditions that warrant specific care.

Beyond the initial assessment, meticulous charting continues throughout the patient's interaction with you. Each intervention performed must be carefully documented, including the rationale behind your choices. For instance, if you administer a medication, note the dosage, route of administration, and the time. This is crucial in monitoring the patient's response to therapy, and in the event of adverse effects, helping identify the cause and take appropriate action. This detailed documentation protects both the patient and yourself legally.

Furthermore, any communication with the patient, their family, or other healthcare professionals needs to be included. If consent was obtained for specific treatments, document this clearly, and be equally diligent if the patient refused any intervention. Any discussions had, the reason behind refusals and any steps taken to address those refusals, are all key aspects. Remember, clarity and completeness is essential to avoid any misunderstandings or misinterpretations.

Thorough documentation goes beyond mere listing of facts; it's about providing context. For instance, a seemingly mundane detail like the patient's clothing might indicate exposure to extreme temperatures or specific hazards. The seemingly insignificant can become critically important, so strive for thoroughness in your descriptions. By focusing on creating a complete record you are providing a comprehensive record that facilitates better patient care.

The information you record must be legible and clearly written, avoiding any ambiguity. Use standardized abbreviations and terminology to maintain consistency. You also need to avoid any subjective interpretation, presenting only objective facts. This objective approach prevents bias and ensures that the chart reflects the events accurately. Remember, your patient chart is a legal document; clarity and accuracy are paramount.

Beyond the clinical details, ensure your charts reflect compliance with ethical standards. Maintain patient confidentiality throughout the entire process, only sharing information with authorized personnel. This ethical behaviour protects the patient's privacy and fosters trust in your services. Remember, maintaining privacy is not just a matter of courtesy; it is a legal requirement, so always keep patient information strictly confidential.

Finally, regular reviews and audits of your charting practices are crucial. This involves self-reflection and peer review, to identify areas for improvement, to ensure consistent adherence to established standards and protocols. Ongoing learning and striving for better practices will reflect on the quality of your work and the well-being of the people you treat. This constant strive for self-improvement is a hallmark of professional paramedic practice.

7 Chapter 7: Ethical & Legal Aspects

Maintaining patient confidentiality is paramount. The Health Insurance Portability and Accountability Act (HIPAA) in the United States, and similar legislation in other countries, strictly regulates the sharing of Protected Health Information (PHI). This includes not only names and addresses, but also diagnoses, treatment details, and even seemingly innocuous information like a patient's employment status, which could potentially be used to identify them. Breaching this confidentiality can lead to severe consequences, both professionally and legally, including fines, loss of license, and even criminal charges. Therefore, sharing patient information should only occur on a need-to-know basis, with appropriate authorization and within the confines of established protocols. Remember, safeguarding patient privacy is not just a legal obligation; it's a cornerstone of trust and a critical aspect of the patient-provider relationship. Never underestimate the importance of discretion, and always adhere to the strictest confidentiality standards. Treat every piece of patient information as highly sensitive and confidential, ensuring you handle it with the utmost care and respect.

Informed consent, or its documented refusal, is a fundamental ethical and legal principle. Before providing any treatment, you must ensure the patient understands the proposed procedure, its risks and benefits, and alternative options. This understanding must be achieved through clear, concise communication, taking into account any language barriers or cognitive impairments. Only then can you obtain genuine informed consent. Should the patient refuse treatment, this refusal must be meticulously documented, including the reason for refusal and any attempts made to persuade the patient otherwise. It is equally crucial to respect the patient's autonomy, even if their decision seems unwise or even potentially harmful. Forcibly administering treatment without proper consent constitutes a serious legal and ethical violation with serious consequences. Remember to clearly communicate options and alternatives. Accurate documentation safeguards everyone involved and highlights the professionalism and ethical integrity you display.

Understanding your scope of practice is critical for both ethical and legal compliance. This scope is defined by your training, licensing, and the specific regulations of your jurisdiction. Exceeding your scope of practice exposes you to liability and potential disciplinary actions. Conversely, failing to provide necessary care within your scope of practice can also have serious legal and ethical implications. Stay updated on any changes in regulations and guidelines, and always practice within the boundaries legally defined for your position. This ensures that you provide safe and effective care while mitigating risks. The importance of continued professional development cannot be overstated. Consistent upskilling is essential, not only for self-improvement but also for fulfilling legal responsibilities within the role. Maintaining a sharp understanding of your scope of practice is crucial for efficient communication with colleagues and for navigating the legal parameters of your profession. Knowing your limits is just as important as knowing your capabilities.

Navigating ethical dilemmas in emergency situations can be challenging. You may encounter situations where resources are scarce, decisions must be made quickly, and the best course of action is not immediately apparent. In these instances, prioritizing patient welfare while adhering to ethical principles is essential. Consider factors such as beneficence (acting in the patient's best interest), non-maleficence (avoiding harm), justice (fair and equitable distribution of resources), and autonomy (respecting patient's choices). Utilize established ethical frameworks and guidelines to guide your decision-making process. Remember, ethical decision-making is a continuous process of reflection and learning, and involving supervisors and colleagues can prove immensely valuable, especially in intricate scenarios. These discussions offer different perspectives and insights, contributing to a more comprehensive and ethical solution. Your aim is to ensure the best possible outcome for every patient, within your legal capabilities. Documenting every decision and its rationale is vital for transparency and protection against future misunderstandings or legal ramifications.

The legal ramifications of negligence can have devastating consequences. Negligence is defined as a failure to provide the standard of care that a reasonably prudent paramedic would have provided in similar circumstances. This failure can result in injury or harm to the patient. Proving negligence typically requires demonstrating a duty of care, breach of that duty, causation (a direct link between the breach and the harm), and damages. To avoid negligence claims, adhere to established protocols and guidelines, document your actions thoroughly, and continuously update your knowledge and skills. Comprehensive documentation and adherence to best practices are crucial to protect you and your team from legal consequences. Regular reviews of procedures and standards of practice, coupled with rigorous ongoing training, ensure that you deliver the highest quality care while limiting legal risks. Being aware of potential legal pitfalls and understanding how to avoid them is paramount to maintaining your professional integrity and protecting yourself in emergency situations. Always strive to provide the highest quality patient care, which will naturally help mitigate against claims of negligence.

7.1 Patient Confidentiality

Maintaining patient confidentiality is paramount, a cornerstone of ethical practice and a legal obligation. Breaching this trust can have severe consequences, both professionally and legally, potentially damaging your reputation and leading to disciplinary action or even lawsuits. Therefore, understanding and upholding confidentiality is not simply a matter of professional courtesy; it's a critical aspect of your job.

Protecting patient information extends beyond simply not gossiping about a case. It encompasses every interaction, from the initial assessment to the final report. This includes written documentation, verbal communication, and even seemingly innocuous actions like leaving patient files visible on a computer screen. Remember, every piece of information a patient shares with you – their medical history, personal details, even the nature of their emergency – is considered confidential. Treat it as such.

The legal framework surrounding patient confidentiality is complex and varies depending on your jurisdiction. However, the core principles remain consistent. Many countries have laws like HIPAA in the US, that specifically protect patient health information. These regulations often define what constitutes protected health information (PHI) and outline strict guidelines for its use and disclosure. Ignorance of these laws is not an excuse for noncompliance. Familiarize yourself with the relevant legislation in your region.

Beyond legal ramifications, there are also significant ethical considerations. Patients trust you with their most vulnerable information, expecting you to handle it with the utmost discretion and respect. This trust is fundamental to the therapeutic relationship and the effective provision of care. Violating that trust can profoundly impact your patient's well-being, potentially causing them emotional distress and further compromising their health. Always remember, the patient's trust is a valuable asset that must be jealously guarded.

So, how do you practically maintain patient confidentiality in the often-chaotic environment of emergency response? First, always be mindful of your surroundings. Avoid discussing patient details in public areas where others might overhear. When documenting patient information, use only secure systems and ensure that all files are properly secured when not in use. Avoid using casual terms or nicknames for patients in your communications; use only the information necessary in your reporting. Be cautious even when seemingly innocuous remarks could accidentally reveal sensitive information.

Furthermore, limit access to patient information to those who have a legitimate need to know. This includes your team members directly involved in the patient's care and any authorized healthcare professionals involved in the subsequent treatment. Strictly avoid disclosing information to family members or friends unless the patient has explicitly given their consent. This can be difficult with emotional family members during stressful situations, but your professional obligation is to the patient's confidentiality. Always err on the side of caution.

Finally, ongoing education is crucial. Confidentiality protocols and regulations evolve, so staying updated is vital. Participate in continuing education programs that address relevant legal and ethical updates. Understand any technology-based improvements to patient data management and make sure your approach aligns with the latest standards and requirements. This proactive approach ensures that you're not only complying with the law but also upholding the highest ethical standards in your practice. Remember, protecting patient confidentiality is not just a job requirement, it's a commitment to the ethical practice of medicine.

7.2 Consent & Refusal

Obtaining informed consent is paramount in emergency medicine. It's not merely a formality; it's a cornerstone of ethical practice and legal protection. This process involves clearly explaining the procedure, its potential benefits and risks, and offering the patient a genuine opportunity to agree or refuse treatment. Remember, a patient's right to self-determination is absolute, even in life-threatening situations. Your role is to provide the necessary information for an informed decision, not to coerce or influence their choice. Documentation is key, meticulously recording the conversation, the patient's understanding, and their expressed wishes.

The concept of capacity is critical. A patient must possess the mental capacity to understand the information presented and weigh the potential consequences of their decision. This capacity can be affected by various factors, including age, mental health conditions, or the effects of medications or injury. If a patient lacks capacity, you must seek consent from their legal guardian or next of kin. However, always strive to involve the patient in the decision-making process to the best extent possible, even if their input is limited. Remember, respecting their dignity is non-negotiable.

Refusal of treatment presents unique challenges. A patient's refusal, even of life-saving treatment, must be respected provided they possess the capacity to make that decision. Thorough documentation is essential in these instances. This involves meticulously recording the patient's refusal, the explanation you provided, and any attempts made to persuade them to reconsider, while always respecting their autonomy. You must be clear and concise in the documentation, emphasizing that all efforts were made to convey the importance of treatment and that the patient's choice was fully understood and accepted.

However, the ethical and legal obligations are nuanced. The right to refuse treatment is not absolute. If a patient is deemed to lack capacity or poses a danger to themselves or others, legally mandated interventions may be necessary. This calls for a thorough understanding of relevant legislation and guidelines. These legal frameworks will help define the boundaries within which you operate. It's imperative to consult with medical control or legal counsel in such complicated situations. Never hesitate to seek assistance, as the well-being of the patient and your legal standing are paramount.

Furthermore, consider the impact of cultural and linguistic barriers. Always ensure clear and effective communication, perhaps using interpreters or translated materials when necessary. Misunderstandings can arise from language differences or cultural variations on the concept of consent. Sensitivity and respect are vital to ensure effective communication. Your objective is to build trust, making it vital to approach the patient with empathy and understanding, while remembering that they are the decision-maker in their healthcare choices.

Dealing with minors requires a different approach. The legal framework surrounding consent for minors varies, often depending on their age and maturity level. In most situations, parental or guardian consent is necessary. However, some jurisdictions recognize a minor's right to consent to certain types of treatment, particularly related to reproductive health or substance abuse. Familiarize yourself with the relevant laws in your region, as the specific rules and procedures will influence your actions. This careful adherence to legal standards is crucial in these delicate situations.

The concept of implied consent plays a crucial role in emergency scenarios. If a patient is unconscious or unable to communicate their wishes, and their life is in immediate danger, implied consent is assumed. This allows you to provide necessary treatment to stabilize their condition. Nevertheless, this is not a carte blanche for intervention. Actions should always be limited to what is strictly necessary to save life or prevent further injury.

Always strive to act in the patient's best interest while respecting their inherent rights.
Ultimately, navigating consent and refusal requires a delicate balance of respect, communication, and knowledge. Understanding the nuances of capacity, documentation, and legal frameworks is essential to responsible and ethical practice. It's your commitment to these principles that safeguards both your patients and your professional reputation. Remember, the aim is not only to deliver appropriate medical care but also to empower patients in controlling their healthcare journey. It's a crucial aspect of building patient trust. Your actions, therefore, must always reflect this balance, guiding your decisions and actions in every encounter.

7.3 Scope of Practice

Understanding your scope of practice is paramount; it's the bedrock upon which your entire career rests. It's not merely a list of allowed procedures; it's a framework for ethical and legal conduct, ensuring both patient safety and your own protection. This understanding prevents you from exceeding your authorized abilities, a serious error with potentially devastating consequences. Ignoring these boundaries could lead to disciplinary actions, legal repercussions, and—worst of all—harm to the very people you're sworn to protect.
Operating within your defined scope means adhering to established protocols and guidelines. This isn't about stifling innovation; it's about prioritizing patient well-being by ensuring interventions are performed by appropriately trained individuals. Your certification and training dictate specific procedures you are qualified to execute, and exceeding these can expose you to significant liability. Always remember that this isn't about personal limitations, it's about a systemic approach to responsible healthcare.
Every state, and even sometimes specific regions within a state,

will have its own slightly varied set of regulations. Therefore, familiarizing yourself with the exact regulations governing your area is non-negotiable. Regularly review your state's paramedic practice act and associated guidelines. These documents outline the specific procedures you're permitted to perform, the medications you may administer, and the circumstances under which you can legally act. Staying updated ensures you are always operating within the bounds of the law, minimizing legal and professional risks. Consider subscribing to newsletters or alerts to receive timely updates on any changes in regulations.

Staying abreast of legal changes and best practices is an ongoing process, not a one-time task. Continuous professional development isn't merely recommended; it's essential. Attending workshops, conferences, and online courses, coupled with reading professional journals, will allow you to refine your skills and stay current with evolving standards. This continuous learning doesn't just improve your practical skills, it demonstrates a commitment to providing the highest level of care, actively reducing professional liability. It is also essential for maintaining your certification.

Knowing your limitations is as important as knowing your skills. Recognizing when a situation exceeds your expertise and requires the intervention of a more specialized medical professional (such as an emergency physician) is crucial. This isn't a sign of weakness; it's a hallmark of responsible practice. Promptly requesting appropriate backup, or transferring care appropriately to more qualified personnel, is a vital aspect of patient-centered care and legal compliance. Never hesitate to seek consultation or additional support when facing a challenging or ambiguous situation.

Effective communication is central to navigating the complexities of scope of practice. Clearly communicating your limitations and the need for additional support to colleagues, supervisors, and other medical professionals is paramount. Vague or ambiguous communication can lead to misunderstandings and potentially disastrous consequences. Use precise and unambiguous language to explain the situation and request assistance when needed. Remember the chain of command. Always know who to contact for support and guidance. Establish and maintain effective communication channels to ensure the safety and well-being of your patient.

Documentation plays a critical role in demonstrating adherence to your scope of practice. Maintaining meticulous records of all your actions, including assessments, interventions, and communications with other healthcare professionals, is essential. This documentation provides a clear and comprehensive account of your involvement in each case, proving your actions were consistent with established protocols and within the legal framework. Thorough and accurate documentation not only protects you legally but also contributes to better patient care by providing a clear timeline of events. Maintain neat, organized records, using standardized forms and avoiding vague or subjective statements.

Finally, remember that your scope of practice is not static. It evolves with your experience, training, and advancement within the profession. As you gain further qualifications, your responsibilities and the range of procedures you are authorized to perform will expand. However, each advancement should be viewed as an opportunity for enhanced proficiency and responsibility, demanding even greater vigilance in adhering to established guidelines and maintaining professional integrity. Consistent self-reflection and professional growth are critical to operating successfully and safely within the ever-evolving paramedic scope of practice. Always stay informed, and always prioritize patient safety.

www.ingramcontent.com/pod-product-compliance
Lightning Source LLC
LaVergne TN
LVHW022025200926
848481LV00007B/2550
* 9 7 9 8 3 4 9 2 8 3 7 1 0 *